Ella (Ulipristal Acetate) vs. Plan B (Levonorgestrel)

Understanding Your Options in Emergency Contraception

Grace O. Williams

Copyright © 2024 by Grace O. Williams

All rights reserved.

No part of this publication may be reproduced, distributed, or transmitted in any form or by any means, including photocopying, recording, or other electronic or mechanical methods, without the prior written permission of the publisher, except in the case of brief quotations embodied in critical reviews and certain other non-commercial uses permitted by copyright law. For permission requests, write to the publisher at the address below.

Table of contents

CHAPTER 1 .... **5**
  INTRODUCTION TO EMERGENCY CONTRACEPTION 5
CHAPTER 2 .... **9**
  HOW THEY WORK: MECHANISMS OF ACTION 9
CHAPTER 3 .... **14**
  EFFECTIVENESS AND SUCCESS RATES 14
CHAPTER 4 .... **19**
  USAGE GUIDELINES AND TIMING 19
CHAPTER 5 .... **24**
  SIDE EFFECTS AND SAFETY PROFILES 24
CHAPTER 6 .... **30**
  BODY WEIGHT AND EFFECTIVENESS 30
CHAPTER 7 .... **36**
  AVAILABILITY AND ACCESSIBILITY 36
CHAPTER 8 .... **42**
  PHARMACOKINETICS AND DRUG INTERACTIONS 42
CHAPTER 9 .... **49**
  MORAL, ETHICAL, AND CULTURAL CONSIDERATIONS 49
CHAPTER 10 .... **55**
  WHO SHOULD USE WHICH? PRACTICAL ADVICE FOR USERS 56
CHAPTER 11 .... **62**

Debunking Myths and Misconceptions 62

CHAPTER 12 ....**69**
Personal Stories and Testimonials 69

CHAPTER 13 ....**77**
Regulatory and Approval History..77

CHAPTER 14 ....**85**
Future of Emergency Contraception...85

CHAPTER 15 ....**94**
A Practical Guide to Using Emergency Contraception 94
   Step 1: Deciding Which Emergency Contraceptive to Use....95
   Step 2: Obtaining the Medication.......................................96
   Step 3: Purchasing and Handling..97
   Step 4: Taking the Medication..97
   Step 5: Managing Side Effects..98
   Step 6: Monitoring Your Menstrual Cycle..........................99
   Step 7: Planning for the Future...99
   Additional Considerations...100
   Handling Special Situations..100

CONCLUSION...**103**
APPENDIX...**110**

Chapter 1

Introduction to Emergency Contraception

"Imagine facing an unexpected situation where you need an emergency solution to avoid an unplanned pregnancy. Ulipristal Acetate and Plan B are here to offer you that peace of mind. But how do you know which one is right for you? Let's explore how these options work and what they mean for your body and your future."

Life can be unpredictable, and sometimes, even with the best plans in place, we encounter moments that require quick and effective decisions. Unprotected sex, missed pills, or contraceptive failures like a broken condom can all lead to unexpected scenarios. In these moments, emergency contraception steps in as a critical tool—a backup plan to prevent pregnancy when things haven't gone as intended.

Emergency contraception (EC) is not about planning or replacing regular contraceptive methods; it is about providing an option when accidents happen. In today's world, there are two main options available—ulipristal acetate (often known as Ella) and levonorgestrel-based pills like Plan B. These medications are designed to give individuals more control over their reproductive health, providing a safe way to prevent pregnancy after unexpected events.

However, as with any medical choice, understanding which option is best for you requires some knowledge. Not all emergency contraceptives are the same—they differ in how they work, how effective they are, when they should be used, and even how they are accessed. For some, the difference between ulipristal acetate and Plan B could mean the difference between success and failure in preventing pregnancy.

In this chapter, we'll lay the foundation for understanding what emergency contraception is, how it differs from regular birth control, and why ulipristal acetate and Plan B have become leading names in this field. We'll also touch on the importance of timing and accessibility, and address some common questions that arise when someone is considering using these drugs.

By the end of this chapter, you will have a solid grasp of what emergency contraception means for you—how it can empower you to take control in situations that otherwise feel beyond your control. We'll aim to demystify these options, providing the essential information you need to make an informed decision about your health and future.

Emergency contraception is not just about preventing pregnancy; it's about empowerment. It is about having options, having knowledge, and having the freedom to choose what is best for your body. Whether you're just learning about these methods for the first time or seeking clarity on which one fits your needs, this guide will walk you through the essentials—making it easier for you to feel confident, secure, and informed.

So, let's get started—because understanding your options today means being better prepared for whatever comes your way tomorrow.

Chapter 2

How They Work: Mechanisms of Action

"Ever wondered what happens in your body when you take emergency contraception? Understanding how ulipristal acetate and Plan B work can empower you to make informed decisions. Let's take a closer look at the science behind preventing pregnancy after unprotected sex."

Emergency contraception might seem like a simple solution—take a pill and reduce the risk of pregnancy—but the truth lies in the complex and fascinating ways these medications interact with the body. To fully understand which option is best for you, it helps to have a grasp of how each one actually prevents pregnancy. The mechanisms behind ulipristal acetate and Plan B are effective but distinct, reflecting the different pathways they use to delay or prevent ovulation.

When you take emergency contraception, it's like giving your body specific instructions to adjust its usual reproductive processes. The primary objective for both ulipristal acetate and Plan B is to prevent ovulation—the release of an egg from the ovary. No egg, no fertilization, no pregnancy. However, the timing, potency, and specific action of each drug differ in important ways, which can significantly affect how successful they are in preventing pregnancy.

Ulipristal acetate works as a selective progesterone receptor modulator. This means it can block the effects of the hormone progesterone, which is essential for ovulation to occur. By doing this, ulipristal acetate effectively delays or stops ovulation even when it's about to happen, giving it an edge over other options if taken later in the cycle. It's designed to work throughout the ovulation process, making it a strong contender when timing is critical.

Plan B, on the other hand, is a high dose of **levonorgestrel**, a synthetic hormone similar to the naturally occurring hormone progesterone. It works mainly by preventing ovulation if taken early enough. If the body has not yet started preparing for ovulation, Plan B can successfully suppress this process. However, it becomes less effective as ovulation approaches because it cannot reliably stop an egg that is already prepared for release.

Another key difference is how each drug interacts with the uterine environment. **Ulipristal acetate** may also alter the endometrium (the lining of the uterus) to prevent a fertilised egg from implanting. While this effect is less well-defined, it's part of what makes ulipristal acetate effective throughout a broader window. **Plan B**, conversely, has limited influence on the uterine lining once ovulation has occurred, which is why it's most effective the earlier it is taken.

Understanding these mechanisms is crucial because it highlights how both drugs work best under specific conditions. Timing is everything—Plan B is most effective in the early stages of the menstrual cycle, whereas ulipristal acetate can offer better protection even when ovulation is imminent. This difference can help you decide which emergency contraceptive is right for you, depending on how much time has passed since unprotected sex and where you are in your cycle.

It's important to note that neither of these options terminate an existing pregnancy. Unlike abortion pills, ulipristal acetate and Plan B work before pregnancy is established, which is why understanding when and how they work is crucial for making an informed decision.

In this chapter, we will break down these complex processes into clear, understandable insights, helping you grasp the science behind emergency contraception. By understanding how these options work in your body, you'll be better prepared to choose the one that best suits your needs and situation. So, let's explore the biological mechanisms that give you control over your reproductive health when you need it most.

Chapter 3

Effectiveness and Success Rates

"Timing is everything when it comes to emergency contraception. How effective are ulipristal acetate and Plan B at different stages after intercourse? Discover the factors that influence their success rates and how you can maximise their effectiveness."

When it comes to emergency contraception, effectiveness is often the top concern. If you find yourself in a situation where you need to prevent an unplanned pregnancy, understanding just how well each option works can give you a sense of control. This chapter dives into the data behind ulipristal acetate and Plan B, comparing their success rates, and helping you understand when each one is most effective.

Ulipristal acetate and Plan B are both designed to reduce the risk of pregnancy after unprotected sex, but their effectiveness hinges largely on **timing**. How soon you take the pill after the incident, where you are in your menstrual cycle, and even individual factors like body weight all come into play in determining how successful these methods will be. The effectiveness of each option isn't just a simple percentage—it's a combination of multiple variables working together.

The **effectiveness window** is one of the critical differences between the two drugs. **Ulipristal acetate** has been shown to remain effective up to **120 hours (5 days)** after unprotected intercourse, with little reduction in success rates within that time frame. This extended window makes ulipristal acetate an appealing choice for those who may not be able to act immediately after the incident. Its ability to delay ovulation even when it's about to occur means that ulipristal acetate offers a robust level of protection regardless of how close you are to ovulating.

Plan B, by contrast, is most effective when taken within **72 hours (3 days)** after unprotected sex, and its effectiveness diminishes the longer you wait. If taken within the first 24 hours, Plan B can be highly effective, but its success rate decreases significantly as time passes. The reason for this decline is tied to the narrow window in which Plan B can successfully prevent ovulation—once the body has begun preparing for ovulation, the pill becomes less reliable.

There's also the matter of **ovulation timing**. If you're close to ovulating or already in the ovulation window, **ulipristal acetate** has a better chance of delaying the process. Plan B is less effective if ovulation is imminent, as it works primarily by preventing the ovary from releasing an egg. This distinction can be critical in determining which option will work best depending on where you are in your menstrual cycle.

Another factor to consider is **body weight**. Research suggests that both ulipristal acetate and Plan B may be less effective in individuals with a higher **Body Mass Index (BMI)**, but this effect is more pronounced with Plan B. For those with a higher BMI, ulipristal acetate is generally recommended as it retains higher efficacy compared to Plan B, whose effectiveness can drop significantly in such cases. Understanding how body weight plays a role in the success rates of these medications can help you make a more informed choice.

Maximizing effectiveness is about more than just choosing the right pill—it's also about **acting quickly** and being aware of the timing. In this chapter, we'll walk through the factors that influence success rates and offer practical advice on how to ensure you're getting the most protection possible. Whether it's understanding the right time to take the pill, knowing how ovulation affects your choices, or considering your own health factors like weight, being informed is key to using emergency contraception effectively.

By the end of this chapter, you'll have a clear understanding of the success rates of both ulipristal acetate and Plan B, and how you can make sure you're using these options at their maximum potential. When faced with a potentially stressful situation, having accurate knowledge can help turn uncertainty into confidence—because, ultimately, timing truly is everything.

Chapter 4

Usage Guidelines and Timing

"Facing a time-sensitive decision can be stressful. How soon do you need to act after unprotected intercourse? Dive into the usage guidelines for ulipristal acetate and Plan B to understand the best time to use each one—and make the most out of your options."

In situations where you need emergency contraception, acting quickly can be crucial. The pressure of needing to make the right decision at the right time can feel overwhelming, especially when you're faced with different choices and a ticking clock. This chapter is dedicated to taking the stress out of this time-sensitive decision by providing you with clear, actionable guidelines for using **ulipristal acetate** and **Plan B** effectively.

Emergency contraception is all about timing. These pills work best when taken as soon as possible after unprotected sex. However, understanding the specific window of effectiveness for both ulipristal acetate and Plan B can make a significant difference in how successful they are at preventing pregnancy. The key lies in acting swiftly while also understanding the time frames each medication offers.

Plan B, a popular choice, is designed to be taken within **72 hours (3 days)** of unprotected intercourse. The sooner you take it, the better it works. Its effectiveness is highest when taken within the first 24 hours and begins to decline each day afterward. While Plan B can still be used up to 72 hours after the event, it's most reliable if taken as soon as possible. The hormone in Plan B, **levonorgestrel**, works by delaying or preventing ovulation, but its effectiveness diminishes the closer you are to ovulation. This is why quick action is so critical.

On the other hand, **ulipristal acetate** offers a longer window of opportunity. It can be taken up to **120 hours (5 days)** after unprotected sex, providing a longer time frame to make a decision. Unlike Plan B, ulipristal acetate maintains a higher level of effectiveness even if you're approaching ovulation, making it a more suitable option if you're unsure of where you are in your cycle or if it's already been a few days. This flexibility can be especially helpful if circumstances prevent you from accessing emergency contraception immediately.

However, just because **ulipristal acetate** allows for a longer delay doesn't mean you should wait. As with all emergency contraceptives, the **earlier** you take it, the higher your chances of success. It's important to remember that while both options work best as soon as possible, ulipristal acetate provides that added assurance if a delay is unavoidable.

Aside from the **timing**, it's also crucial to understand the **specific guidelines** for using each medication.

Plan B is available over the counter in many countries, making it accessible without a prescription, which can be a major advantage if you need it quickly. **Ulipristal acetate**, on the other hand, often requires a prescription, which can create an extra step in the process of obtaining it. Knowing this ahead of time can help you decide which option to seek based on your circumstances and the availability in your area.

This chapter will also explore **common scenarios** and provide guidance on how to approach them. For example, what should you do if you've already ovulated, or if you're unsure about your cycle? What if it's been more than three days since unprotected sex? We will break down these situations and guide you through the decision-making process, so you can feel confident in your choice.

Finally, we'll touch on **repeat use**—can you use emergency contraception more than once in the same cycle? What are the potential impacts on your menstrual cycle, and what should you know if this isn't the first time you're using it? Understanding these nuances can help you navigate emergency contraception without unnecessary stress or confusion.

By the end of this chapter, you'll know the best time to take **ulipristal acetate** and **Plan B** based on your unique situation. You'll also understand how to use these options effectively, ensuring you're making the most of the emergency contraception available to you. When faced with a time-sensitive decision, knowledge can be your most powerful ally—empowering you to act decisively and with confidence.

Chapter 5

Side Effects and Safety Profiles

"No medication comes without side effects. Knowing what to expect helps you prepare and manage your health effectively. Let's uncover the possible side effects of ulipristal acetate and Plan B and how you can stay safe while using them."

Taking emergency contraception is often a significant decision, one made under pressing circumstances, and it's natural to wonder about its potential side effects. Whether it's **ulipristal acetate** or **Plan B**, understanding how these medications might affect your body can help you feel more in control and better prepared for what's to come. This chapter focuses on the **safety profiles** of both drugs, discussing common side effects, safety concerns, and practical advice on managing them.

Emergency contraceptives are designed to be safe for most individuals, and millions of people around the world have used them without serious complications. However, like any medication, both **ulipristal acetate** and **Plan B** can have side effects. These effects can vary depending on individual factors, including your health, your menstrual cycle, and how your body reacts to hormones. Knowing what to expect can make the experience less intimidating and more manageable.

Let's begin by looking at **ulipristal acetate**. The most commonly reported side effects include **headache**, **abdominal pain**, **nausea**, and **fatigue**. Some people may also experience **dizziness** or **breast tenderness**. These side effects are usually mild and temporary, resolving on their own after a few days. Another notable impact of ulipristal acetate is on your menstrual cycle—it may cause your next period to be **delayed** or **earlier** than usual, and some people may notice a heavier or lighter flow. These changes are generally not cause for concern, but understanding them in advance can help you avoid unnecessary stress.

Plan B shares some similar side effects, such as **nausea, vomiting, dizziness,** and **fatigue**. You might also experience **menstrual changes**—your period may come earlier or later, and its intensity can vary. Some users report **spotting** or **bleeding** between periods after taking Plan B. These changes are a normal reaction to the high dose of levonorgestrel, the hormone used in Plan B, and they do not indicate any long-term issues. It's also worth noting that if you vomit shortly after taking Plan B, you may need to take another dose, as your body may not have had enough time to absorb the medication.

While these side effects are typically not serious, it's important to know when you should seek medical attention. If you experience **severe abdominal pain**, it could be a sign of an ectopic pregnancy, a rare but serious condition where a fertilised egg implants outside the uterus. This condition requires immediate medical intervention. Although ectopic pregnancies are uncommon, recognising the symptoms early can make all the difference in ensuring your safety.

Another aspect to consider is **allergies**. Both ulipristal acetate and Plan B contain inactive ingredients that could cause an allergic reaction in some individuals. If you have known allergies to any medication ingredients, it's crucial to read the labels or consult a healthcare provider before use. Signs of an allergic reaction may include **rash, itching, swelling,** or **difficulty breathing**—symptoms that warrant immediate medical attention.

Drug interactions are another important part of the safety profile of emergency contraceptives. Certain medications can reduce the effectiveness of both ulipristal acetate and Plan B. These include some **antiepileptic drugs, HIV medications**, and even **herbal supplements** like **St. John's Wort.** If you're on any regular medication, it's wise to speak with a healthcare provider to ensure that there won't be any adverse interactions that could compromise the effectiveness of your emergency contraception.

In this chapter, we will also provide practical **tips for managing side effects**. Simple steps like **taking the pill with food** can help minimize nausea, and staying hydrated can help manage symptoms like fatigue or dizziness. Understanding your body's response and knowing what to expect can significantly ease the experience.

It's also essential to address any **emotional effects**. Using emergency contraception can be a stressful experience, and some individuals report feeling anxious or emotional after taking the pill. Understanding that these feelings are normal and temporary can help you navigate the emotional side of this journey more comfortably. If anxiety or worry becomes overwhelming, reaching out to a trusted friend or healthcare provider can offer reassurance and support.

By understanding the **side effects and safety profiles** of ulipristal acetate and Plan B, you can take these medications with greater confidence, knowing what to expect and how to respond to any challenges. This knowledge not only helps you prepare physically but also emotionally, giving you the power to stay informed and in control during what might otherwise be a stressful situation. After all, being aware of how these emergency options affect your body is a key part of using them effectively and safely.

Chapter 6

Body Weight and Effectiveness

"Did you know that your weight might affect how well emergency contraception works? Let's explore how body weight can influence the effectiveness of both ulipristal acetate and Plan B, and what you need to know if BMI is a concern."

When it comes to emergency contraception, there's an often overlooked factor that could significantly influence its effectiveness—**body weight**. Just as each person's body responds differently to medications, weight can play a crucial role in determining how well emergency contraceptive pills work. For those with a higher **Body Mass Index (BMI)**, the effectiveness of **Plan B** and **ulipristal acetate** may vary, which makes understanding these differences essential for making an informed decision.

In this chapter, we will take a closer look at the link between **body weight** and the success rates of **emergency contraceptives**. Knowing how your body may impact the effectiveness of these medications helps ensure that you choose the method that gives you the best possible chance of preventing an unplanned pregnancy.

Plan B, which contains **levonorgestrel**, has been studied extensively, and there is evidence suggesting that its effectiveness may decrease as body weight or BMI increases. Research indicates that Plan B is less effective in individuals weighing more than **165 pounds (75 kg)**, and its success rate significantly drops for those over **175 pounds (79 kg)**. This means that if your weight falls within this range, there is an increased risk that Plan B might not work as effectively as intended. The reason behind this reduced efficacy is likely related to how the body metabolises the hormone levonorgestrel—higher body weight may lead to lower concentrations of the hormone in the bloodstream, thereby reducing its ability to prevent ovulation.

Ulipristal acetate, on the other hand, appears to be less affected by body weight compared to Plan B. Studies show that **ulipristal acetate** is generally more effective for individuals with a higher BMI, maintaining its effectiveness better than levonorgestrel-based pills. However, even with ulipristal acetate, there is some evidence that its efficacy may still be reduced in individuals with significantly higher BMIs, although the reduction is not as pronounced as with Plan B. This makes ulipristal acetate a more reliable option for those concerned about weight affecting the success of their emergency contraception.

If you fall into a higher weight category, this information is particularly important. It doesn't mean that Plan B or ulipristal acetate won't work for you—it simply means you need to be aware of the potential reduction in effectiveness. In some cases, healthcare providers may recommend **other forms of emergency contraception**, such as the **copper intrauterine device (IUD)**, which is highly effective regardless of body weight and can be used up to five days after unprotected sex.

Understanding these nuances is key to making an informed decision that aligns with your body's needs. **Timing** also plays a role—regardless of body weight, taking emergency contraception as soon as possible after unprotected intercourse maximises its effectiveness. If you're concerned about weight impacting the success of your chosen method, speaking with a healthcare provider can provide additional guidance and help you explore the best option for you.

In this chapter, we'll also look at **practical advice** for those concerned about body weight. This includes understanding the best timing for taking emergency contraception, knowing when an alternative method like the copper IUD might be more suitable, and considering how to advocate for your health when discussing emergency contraception with a healthcare professional. It's about making sure that every individual, regardless of size, has the information needed to effectively prevent an unplanned pregnancy.

Body weight is just one of many factors that can influence the effectiveness of emergency contraception, but it's an important one. By understanding how ulipristal acetate and Plan B perform differently based on weight, you can make a more confident choice. Whether that means opting for ulipristal acetate, considering an IUD, or consulting with a healthcare provider for personalised advice, this knowledge empowers you to make the best decision for your health.

By the end of this chapter, you'll have a clearer picture of how body weight may affect the success of emergency contraception and how to navigate your options accordingly. After all, emergency contraception is about providing you with control and confidence in preventing pregnancy—and knowing what works best for your body is a vital part of that journey.

Chapter 7

Availability and Accessibility

"Access to contraception can vary depending on where you live, your financial situation, or your healthcare provider. Find out how easy it is to get your hands on ulipristal acetate and Plan B, and what you need to consider in terms of cost and availability."

When you need **emergency contraception**, time is of the essence, and knowing how and where to access it can make all the difference. However, getting hold of **ulipristal acetate** or **Plan B** isn't always straightforward. The availability of these options can vary widely depending on your location, healthcare system, and financial resources, creating barriers that can make an already stressful situation even more challenging.

This chapter is dedicated to breaking down the **availability and accessibility** of ulipristal acetate and Plan B, helping you understand what factors come into play when trying to obtain these crucial medications. We'll explore the differences between these two contraceptives in terms of how they can be acquired—whether it's over-the-counter, by prescription, or through other channels.

Plan B, also known as the **morning-after pill**, is typically the more accessible of the two options. In many countries, including the United States, Plan B can be purchased **over-the-counter** without a prescription. This ease of access is a significant advantage, especially in situations where every hour counts. You can often find Plan B at local pharmacies, big-box stores, and even some convenience stores, which makes it a convenient option for most people. However, the cost can vary depending on where you buy it. Prices typically range from **$35 to $50**, which may be a barrier for some individuals, particularly those without health insurance or those facing financial difficulties.

In contrast, **ulipristal acetate** (sold under the brand name **Ella**) often requires a **prescription**, which can add an extra layer of complexity to obtaining it. This requirement means you'll need to either visit a healthcare provider or use an online telehealth service to get a prescription, which can take valuable time. On the positive side, ulipristal acetate is generally available at most pharmacies once you have a prescription, but its **cost** can be higher than Plan B, often ranging from **$40 to $60 or more**. Some health insurance plans cover ulipristal acetate, which can help offset the cost, but this depends on your provider and coverage.

Another aspect of **accessibility** is the **regional differences** in availability. In some countries, access to emergency contraception is heavily regulated, which can limit the options available to you. For instance, while Plan B may be available without a prescription in many Western countries, other regions may impose stricter controls, requiring prescriptions or even completely restricting access. Ulipristal acetate, being a relatively newer option, might not be as widely available globally, further limiting choices for individuals in certain areas. Understanding the regulations in your country or region is crucial to knowing what options you have when the need arises.

There's also the consideration of **healthcare support**. If you live in an area with limited healthcare facilities or face challenges accessing a healthcare provider—due to distance, cost, or availability—getting a prescription for ulipristal acetate might not be practical. In such cases, Plan B's over-the-counter status becomes an invaluable advantage. **Telehealth services** have made strides in bridging some of these gaps, allowing people to consult with healthcare providers online and obtain a prescription without an in-person visit, but this solution depends on internet access and regional telehealth regulations.

For those facing **financial constraints**, there are potential solutions. Some clinics, such as **Planned Parenthood**, may offer emergency contraception at a reduced cost or even for free based on income. In some regions, government programs or nonprofit organisations may provide vouchers or assistance to cover the cost of emergency contraceptives. Knowing about these resources in advance can make a huge difference when you're in need.

In this chapter, we will also discuss **privacy** concerns. For some people, privacy is an important consideration when accessing emergency contraception. Purchasing Plan B over the counter may feel less invasive than consulting with a healthcare provider for ulipristal acetate, especially if you prefer to keep your decisions private. Understanding what each option entails—both in terms of how you acquire it and who might be involved—can help you choose the method that feels most comfortable for you.

By the end of this chapter, you'll have a clearer picture of how to access **ulipristal acetate** and **Plan B**, including what to expect in terms of **cost**, **availability**, and **potential barriers**. You'll be better prepared to navigate these challenges, whether it's understanding how to get a prescription, exploring cost-saving options, or knowing where to go for immediate access. Ultimately, having this knowledge beforehand ensures that when you need emergency contraception, you can act swiftly and confidently, without unnecessary delays or obstacles.

Chapter 8

Pharmacokinetics and Drug Interactions

"What happens inside your body after you take emergency contraception? How do other medications affect their efficacy? Understanding the pharmacokinetics and drug interactions can help you make the safest choice for your health."

When you take an emergency contraceptive, a complex set of processes begins within your body. These processes—known collectively as **pharmacokinetics**—determine how the medication is absorbed, distributed, metabolized, and ultimately excreted. Understanding these steps can provide valuable insight into how emergency contraception works and how effective it is at preventing pregnancy. In this chapter, we'll explore what happens after you take **ulipristal acetate** or **Plan B**, and why it matters for making an informed choice.

Pharmacokinetics is a term that might sound technical, but at its core, it simply describes the journey a drug takes through your body. It starts the moment you swallow the pill. First, the drug is **absorbed** into your bloodstream through your gastrointestinal tract, after which it is **distributed** throughout your body to reach its target organs—primarily your reproductive system. There, the active ingredients work to **delay ovulation** and, in some cases, alter the conditions of your uterus to reduce the likelihood of pregnancy.

For **Plan B**, which contains **levonorgestrel**, the goal is to prevent the ovary from releasing an egg. Once ingested, levonorgestrel is rapidly absorbed and reaches its peak concentration in the blood within a few hours. It is then metabolised in the liver and excreted primarily through urine. Because it acts quickly, taking Plan B as soon as possible is crucial to maximise its effectiveness. The pharmacokinetics of Plan B mean that it is most effective during the earlier stages of your cycle—before ovulation has occurred.

Ulipristal acetate, the active ingredient in **Ella**, follows a slightly different path. As a **selective progesterone receptor modulator**, ulipristal acetate binds to progesterone receptors in your body, effectively blocking the hormone's action and delaying ovulation even when it is already in progress. It takes a bit longer to reach its peak concentration compared to Plan B, but its ability to modulate progesterone gives it an extended window of effectiveness—up to five days after unprotected sex. Ulipristal acetate is also metabolised by the liver and then excreted through both urine and faeces.

One key aspect of pharmacokinetics is the potential for **drug interactions**. Both ulipristal acetate and Plan B can be affected by other medications you may be taking. Certain drugs can alter the way emergency contraceptives are **metabolised**, potentially reducing their effectiveness. For example, medications that induce liver enzymes—specifically **cytochrome P450 3A4 (CYP3A4)**—can speed up the breakdown of emergency contraceptives, lowering their concentration in the blood and thus reducing their ability to prevent pregnancy.

Some of the medications that can interfere with the efficacy of both **ulipristal acetate** and **Plan B** include:

- **Antiepileptic drugs** like phenytoin, carbamazepine, and phenobarbital.
- **Rifampin**, an antibiotic used to treat tuberculosis.
- **HIV medications**, such as efavirenz.
- **St. John's Wort**, an herbal supplement often used for mood regulation.

If you are taking any of these medications, it's important to consult with a healthcare provider before relying on emergency contraception. In such cases, your healthcare provider might suggest using a

copper IUD as an alternative form of emergency contraception, as its efficacy is not impacted by these drug interactions.

Additionally, **ulipristal acetate** and **hormonal contraceptives** can interact in a way that reduces their effectiveness. Because ulipristal acetate affects progesterone receptors, taking it too close to regular hormonal contraceptives (like birth control pills, patches, or injections) can reduce the effectiveness of both. It is generally recommended to wait at least **five days** after taking ulipristal acetate before resuming hormonal contraceptives, to ensure that their effectiveness is not compromised.

It's also important to note that emergency contraceptives themselves can impact your **menstrual cycle**. Both ulipristal acetate and Plan B can cause temporary changes such as **delayed periods**, **spotting**, or **heavier menstrual bleeding**. These changes are usually harmless but can sometimes lead to confusion or concern if you're not expecting them. Understanding that these effects are a normal part of how the drug works in your body can help alleviate anxiety and ensure you know when to seek medical advice.

In this chapter, we will also discuss **practical steps** for managing potential drug interactions and ensuring that your emergency contraceptive works as intended. This includes checking the medications or supplements you're currently taking, consulting with a healthcare provider if needed, and considering alternative methods of emergency contraception if drug interactions are likely to be an issue.

By understanding the **pharmacokinetics** of ulipristal acetate and Plan B, you can better appreciate how these medications work within your body, and by being aware of potential **drug interactions**, you can take steps to ensure that you're using emergency contraception safely and effectively. This knowledge empowers you to make informed choices that best support your reproductive health, even when faced with unexpected situations.

Chapter 9

Moral, Ethical, and Cultural Considerations

"Emergency contraception isn't just a medical topic; it's often wrapped in moral, cultural, and ethical discussions. How do these aspects impact your choices, and what do they mean for access and acceptance of these medications? Let's explore these nuanced perspectives."

When discussing **emergency contraception**, it's impossible to ignore the broader societal context in which it exists. Unlike other forms of contraception, emergency contraceptives like **ulipristal acetate** and **Plan B** often spark heated discussions beyond their medical function. These debates involve questions about morality, ethics, cultural beliefs, and even politics. Understanding these perspectives can help you better navigate your own choices, and it also sheds light on why access to emergency contraception can vary so greatly depending on where you are.

One of the core **ethical considerations** surrounding emergency contraception is whether it constitutes a form of **abortion**. While medical science clearly defines emergency contraception as a means to prevent pregnancy—working before fertilisation or implantation occurs—misunderstandings persist. Some individuals and groups argue that any interference with the possibility of conception, especially in the case of **ulipristal acetate**, which might affect the uterine lining, equates to terminating a pregnancy. It's important to clarify that both **Plan B** and **ulipristal acetate** work **before pregnancy is established**, and neither is capable of terminating an existing pregnancy.

These **ethical debates** are often rooted in personal beliefs about when life begins. For those who believe that life starts at conception, emergency contraception may be viewed unfavourably, which affects both individual choices and broader societal attitudes toward these medications. Understanding this can help you make sense of why some regions, organisations, or even healthcare providers may restrict access to emergency contraception or treat it with greater scrutiny.

Cultural perspectives also play a significant role in shaping attitudes towards emergency contraception. In some cultures, there's a strong emphasis on **traditional family values**, which may discourage the use of emergency contraceptives. The use of such methods can be seen as a sign of promiscuity or irresponsibility, especially for unmarried women. This stigma can deter people from seeking emergency contraception even when they need it, fearing judgment from healthcare professionals, pharmacists, or even family members. The result is that many people might not use these vital options due to the fear of social repercussions.

On the other hand, in cultures with more progressive attitudes toward **sexual health**, emergency contraception is viewed as an important component of reproductive rights. It empowers individuals, particularly women, to have more control over their bodies and their futures. For these societies, the emphasis is on **autonomy**, **education**, and ensuring that everyone has access to the resources they need to make informed decisions about their reproductive health. This contrast highlights how deeply cultural beliefs impact the availability and acceptance of emergency contraceptives.

The **political landscape** also plays a major role in shaping access to emergency contraception. In some countries, policies are influenced heavily by religious or moral views, which can result in restrictive laws or lack of availability. For example, **ulipristal acetate** might not be available in certain regions due to its classification or the ethical debates surrounding its mechanism of action. Meanwhile, **Plan B** may be available over the counter in some places but require a prescription in others, depending on the local regulatory stance on contraception. These variations can make accessing emergency contraception a challenge that extends far beyond simply visiting a pharmacy.

It's also important to address the **role of religion**. In many communities, religious teachings significantly influence individual choices regarding contraception. Some faiths advocate against any form of birth control, while others may permit the use of contraception but oppose emergency options like Plan B or ulipristal acetate. For individuals whose personal beliefs are closely tied to religious doctrine, making a decision about whether to use emergency contraception can be deeply complex and emotionally charged. This highlights the need for compassionate, **nonjudgmental healthcare** and comprehensive education that respects individual beliefs while providing accurate information.

Education and awareness are key factors in overcoming the moral and cultural barriers surrounding emergency contraception. When people have access to clear, scientifically accurate information, they are better equipped to understand what these medications are and what they are not. Education can also dispel myths and reduce stigma, encouraging people to make choices that are best for their health without undue influence from misinformation or societal pressure.

we'll also explore how different countries and cultures handle **public health campaigns** around emergency contraception. In some regions, efforts to educate the public about emergency contraception are robust, aiming to empower individuals with knowledge and resources. In other areas, silence or misinformation prevails, contributing to the continued stigma and limited use of these important medications. Understanding these differences provides a broader picture of why access can be straightforward in some places and fraught with obstacles in others.

By delving into the **moral, ethical, and cultural considerations** of emergency contraception, this chapter aims to provide you with a well-rounded understanding of the broader context in which these medications exist. Whether you are personally navigating these considerations or seeking to understand why such a simple medical option can be so controversial, having a nuanced perspective helps demystify the debate and brings clarity to your own choices.

Ultimately, emergency contraception is more than just a medical tool—it's a representation of individual autonomy, cultural norms, ethical beliefs, and societal attitudes. By understanding these interconnected aspects, you can make informed decisions that align with both your health needs and your personal values.

Chapter 10

Who Should Use Which? Practical Advice for Users

"With two options available, which one is the best for you? From timing to personal health conditions, learn how to make the choice between ulipristal acetate and Plan B, tailored to your unique situation."

Choosing the right **emergency contraceptive** can feel overwhelming, especially when you're in a situation that requires quick action. With **ulipristal acetate** and **Plan B** both offering effective ways to prevent pregnancy, how do you decide which one is best for you? The answer depends on a number of factors—timing, body weight, your health conditions, and even personal preferences.

In this chapter, we'll guide you through the practical considerations that can help you choose between these two emergency contraceptives. Understanding the unique benefits and limitations of **ulipristal acetate** and **Plan B** will allow you to make an informed choice that aligns with your specific needs and circumstances.

One of the most important factors to consider is **timing**. If you've had unprotected sex or experienced contraceptive failure, time is a crucial element in determining which option is best for you. **Plan B** is most effective when taken within **72 hours (3 days)**, and its efficacy decreases as more time passes. **Ulipristal acetate**, however, provides a longer window of opportunity—up to **120 hours (5 days)**—without losing much of its effectiveness over that time. This means that if it has been more than three days since the incident, ulipristal acetate is generally the more reliable choice.

Ovulation timing is another key consideration. **Plan B** works by preventing ovulation, but if you are close to or already ovulating, its effectiveness may be significantly reduced. **Ulipristal acetate**, on the other hand, can still delay ovulation even when it is imminent, giving it an edge if you're unsure of where you are in your cycle. If you believe ovulation is close, ulipristal acetate is likely the better option.

Your **body weight** can also play a role in determining which emergency contraceptive is most effective. Studies suggest that **Plan B** may be less effective for individuals with a **Body Mass Index (BMI)** above **25**. If you weigh more than **165 pounds (75 kg)**, Plan B's success rate may decline, whereas **ulipristal acetate** tends to maintain its effectiveness across a broader range of body weights. For those with a higher BMI, ulipristal acetate is generally the preferred choice.

Health conditions and medications you are taking are also crucial factors to consider. Some medications, including certain **antiepileptics**, HIV

medications, and even **St. John's Wort**, can reduce the effectiveness of both Plan B and ulipristal acetate. If you are taking any medication that could interfere with emergency contraception, consulting a healthcare provider is essential. In some cases, they may recommend an alternative, such as the **copper IUD**, which is not affected by these interactions and is highly effective.

Another aspect to consider is **accessibility. Plan B** is often available over the counter in pharmacies, making it a more convenient option if you need emergency contraception quickly and without a prescription. **Ulipristal acetate**, on the other hand, typically requires a prescription, which might make accessing it more challenging depending on your situation. If you need immediate access and don't have a prescription, Plan B may be the more practical option despite its limitations in certain conditions. However, in some areas, **telehealth services** may provide a quick way to obtain a prescription for ulipristal acetate, so it's worth checking your options.

Menstrual cycle considerations also come into play. Both **ulipristal acetate** and **Plan B** can alter your menstrual cycle—causing your period to come earlier or later, or changing the intensity of your flow. While these changes are typically harmless, they can be confusing, especially if you're concerned about a potential pregnancy. Understanding that these side effects are common and temporary can help you decide which option feels more manageable for you.

Lastly, it's worth considering **personal comfort and preference**. For some individuals, taking a pill without needing to consult a doctor feels more comfortable, which might make **Plan B** more appealing due to its over-the-counter availability. Others might prefer **ulipristal acetate** for its longer window of effectiveness and better success rate under certain conditions, even if it requires obtaining a prescription. Knowing what makes you feel most comfortable and empowered in making this decision is just as important as the medical aspects.

In this chapter, we also present **scenarios** to help illustrate how these factors come together in real-life situations. Whether you're dealing with a condom failure late in your cycle, worried about ovulation timing, or need a backup plan after missed contraceptive pills, these examples will provide a clear, practical guide to help you choose the right option.

By the end of this chapter, you'll have a thorough understanding of when to choose **ulipristal acetate** versus **Plan B**, based on your unique circumstances. This information will enable you to make the best choice for your body, ensuring that you have the control and confidence needed when facing an unexpected situation. After all, emergency contraception is about giving you the power to manage your reproductive health effectively, and knowing which option suits your needs is key to making that happen.

Chapter 11

Debunking Myths and Misconceptions

"There's a lot of misinformation floating around about emergency contraception. Are these drugs forms of abortion? Do they cause long-term damage? Let's separate the myths from the facts and empower you with the truth."

Emergency contraception, while widely used and medically validated, remains a topic surrounded by myths and misunderstandings. Whether it's confusion about how these medications work or misconceptions about their safety, misinformation can cause unnecessary fear and deter people from making informed choices. In this chapter, we aim to debunk some of the most common myths surrounding **ulipristal acetate** and **Plan B**, giving you the facts you need to make confident decisions about your health.

One of the most pervasive myths is that **emergency contraceptives** are the same as **abortion pills**. This misunderstanding stems from a lack of clarity about how these medications work. Both **Plan B** and **ulipristal acetate** are designed to prevent pregnancy **before** it occurs, by delaying or preventing ovulation. If there is no egg released, there can be no fertilisation, and thus, no pregnancy. Neither drug can terminate an existing pregnancy. In contrast, **abortion pills** like **mifepristone** and **misoprostol** are used to end an established pregnancy. Understanding this key distinction is crucial for dispelling the false narrative that emergency contraception is a form of abortion.

Another widespread myth is that using **emergency contraception** will cause **long-term damage** to your reproductive health or fertility. This is simply not true. Numerous studies have shown that **ulipristal**

acetate and **Plan B** do not have any lasting effects on fertility. After using emergency contraception, your menstrual cycle may be temporarily altered—you may experience a delayed or earlier period, but these changes are short-lived. Once your next cycle begins, your fertility returns to normal. This means you can become pregnant again as soon as your body ovulates, so it's important to continue using regular contraception if you want to prevent pregnancy in the future.

There is also a myth that **emergency contraception** is less effective or dangerous if used **multiple times**. While emergency contraception is not meant to replace regular birth control methods, it is safe to use more than once if needed. The occasional use of **ulipristal acetate** or **Plan B** does not pose significant health risks. However, relying on these methods frequently is less effective than using a consistent form of birth control, like the pill, IUD, or condoms. The key is to see emergency contraception as a backup method rather than your primary form of birth control. Frequent use can lead to more **irregular menstrual cycles**, but it does not cause harm or reduce your chances of getting pregnant in the future.

Some people believe that **emergency contraceptives** don't work for individuals who have already **ovulated**. While this is partially true for **Plan B**, which is less effective once ovulation has begun, **ulipristal acetate** can still work by delaying ovulation even if it's about to happen. This makes ulipristal acetate a more reliable choice if you are unsure of your cycle timing or if you are close to ovulating. Understanding this difference between the two options can help you make a better-informed decision based on where you are in your cycle.

A common myth is that **emergency contraception** is only for **teenagers** or **unmarried women**, leading to unnecessary stigma. In reality, emergency contraception is for **anyone** who is at risk of an unplanned pregnancy and needs an effective backup plan. Whether you're in a long-term relationship, married, or in your twenties or forties, these medications are designed to provide a solution when your regular contraceptive method fails, or in cases of unprotected intercourse. Breaking down this stereotype is essential for normalising the use of emergency contraception as part of responsible sexual health.

There are also fears that **emergency contraceptives** can cause serious side effects or health complications. While it's true that side effects like **nausea**, **headaches**, or **menstrual changes** can occur, these are typically mild and temporary. Neither **Plan B** nor **ulipristal acetate** is associated with any serious long-term health risks. For most people, these side effects will subside within a few days, and their overall impact on health is minimal. In rare cases where side effects persist or worsen, it's always a good idea to consult a healthcare provider, but the likelihood of lasting harm is extremely low.

Another misconception is that **emergency contraception** is 100% effective. While these medications significantly reduce the risk of pregnancy, they are not infallible. **Plan B** is about **87% effective** when taken within the first 72 hours, and **ulipristal acetate** is up to **95% effective** when taken within 120 hours. The sooner you take them, the higher the chances of success, but no method is completely guaranteed. Factors like **timing**, **body weight**, and **ovulation status** can influence how well the drug works. It's important to understand that emergency contraception is a highly effective backup, but it is not foolproof.

We also address the myth that **emergency contraception** is difficult to access or obtain. While availability can vary depending on where you live, in many countries, **Plan B** is available over the counter without a prescription, making it relatively easy to access. **Ulipristal acetate** often requires a prescription, but **telehealth services** have made it easier to obtain one quickly if you need it. Awareness of your local resources, pharmacies, and online services can help you avoid the stress of searching for emergency contraception when you need it most.

By the end of this chapter, you'll have a clear understanding of the **facts** surrounding **ulipristal acetate** and **Plan B**, leaving behind the myths that cloud these vital options. Separating **truth** from **misinformation** will empower you to make informed choices with confidence, free from unnecessary fear or doubt. Emergency contraception is a safe, effective way to prevent unplanned pregnancies, and by understanding how it really works, you can take charge of your reproductive health with the knowledge you need.

Chapter 12

Personal Stories and Testimonials

"Real stories can bring comfort, understanding, and even clarity. Hear from individuals who've used ulipristal acetate or Plan B—how they made their choice, what their experiences were like, and what they learned from the process."

Deciding to use **emergency contraception** can be a deeply personal experience. It often comes during a time of uncertainty, stress, or fear—moments when things didn't go as planned. During these times, it can be immensely helpful to hear from others who have walked the same path, faced the same decisions, and emerged with their own insights. This chapter is dedicated to sharing the **real stories** of individuals who've used **ulipristal acetate** or **Plan B**, providing an honest look at their experiences, challenges, and reflections.

There's something powerful about listening to real voices. Scientific facts and guidelines are important, but **personal stories** add depth and bring the information to life. Through the narratives of others, you may find similarities to your own situation, which can offer comfort and help you feel less alone in your experience. Whether it's a story of using emergency contraception after a contraceptive failure or a narrative about the anxiety of waiting for a delayed period, these experiences provide insights that are invaluable, particularly when you need reassurance or understanding.

We start with **Emily**, a college student who had to make a quick decision after a condom failure. She shares how she initially felt panicked and unsure about what to do, but the availability of **Plan B** over the counter at her local pharmacy provided her with some peace of mind. Emily talks about her concerns regarding potential side effects and how she ultimately felt relieved once she took the pill. Her story emphasizes the importance of having immediate access to emergency contraception and how that availability helped her regain a sense of control during a stressful moment.

Next, we hear from **Sophia**, who chose **ulipristal acetate** after realising she was likely close to ovulating when her contraceptive method failed. Sophia's story sheds light on the decision-making process involved in choosing the right emergency contraceptive. She describes her consultation with a healthcare provider, who recommended ulipristal acetate for its higher effectiveness during ovulation. Sophia explains the prescription process, the slight delay in getting the medication, and how she managed her anxiety during that time. For Sophia, the key takeaway was the importance of having access to reliable medical information and the value of talking to a healthcare professional who could guide her.

Mia, a mother of two, shares her experience of using **Plan B** after missing her regular birth control pill. As a working mom, Mia was juggling a lot and missed a few days of her pill schedule, which led to an unplanned risk. Her story highlights the practical considerations of being a busy parent and the challenges of keeping up with birth control while managing daily responsibilities. She talks about the mild side effects she experienced, like nausea and a delayed period, and how understanding what to expect helped her stay calm. Mia's story provides insight into how emergency contraception can be a necessary safety net, even for those who already use regular birth control.

We also hear from **Alex**, a transgender man, who shares his unique perspective on accessing **emergency contraception**. For Alex, the decision to use ulipristal acetate was challenging due to concerns about judgment and misunderstandings at the pharmacy. His story speaks to the emotional hurdles that some individuals face, particularly those in the

LGBTQ+ community, when trying to access reproductive healthcare. Alex ultimately used a telehealth service to get his prescription, which made the process easier and more comfortable. His story underscores the importance of inclusive healthcare and the barriers that still need to be broken down to ensure everyone has equal access to emergency contraception.

Hannah recounts her experience using **Plan B** twice within a year, after two separate incidents where her primary contraception failed. Hannah's story highlights the misconceptions around using emergency contraception multiple times. Initially, she worried about the impact on her body or future fertility, but after researching and talking with her doctor, she learned that using Plan B more than once is safe. Hannah's experience reassured her that she wasn't harming her reproductive health, and it also motivated her to switch to a more consistent birth control method that better suited her lifestyle.

Daniela, a young professional, talks about her experience with **ulipristal acetate** when she was travelling abroad. She describes the difficulties she faced in trying to find the medication in a country where it was less readily available and how she managed to eventually get a prescription. Daniela's story is a testament to the challenges of accessing emergency contraception in different regions and how planning ahead—even when travelling—can make a significant difference.

Lastly, we include the story of **Erica**, who felt a lot of anxiety after taking **Plan B** due to the stigma she felt from friends and even her pharmacist. Erica's experience highlights the **emotional impact** that can come with using emergency contraception, especially when judgment is involved. Despite the stress, Erica reflects on how having access to this option allowed her to make the best decision for herself at that moment. Her story helps us understand that while the physical aspects of taking emergency contraception are important, the emotional experience can be equally significant.

These stories provide a human element that goes beyond medical facts. They illustrate the **diverse situations** in which emergency contraception becomes necessary and the **real-life challenges** that people face—from navigating pharmacies to understanding which option is best for them. Whether it's a story of feeling empowered, navigating uncertainty, or managing side effects, each experience brings a valuable perspective to the conversation about **ulipristal acetate** and **Plan B**.

By sharing these **personal testimonials**, we aim to provide a source of comfort and clarity for those who may find themselves in similar circumstances. Every story is different, but they all reflect a common goal—taking control of one's reproductive health when the unexpected happens. Through these narratives, we hope you gain a deeper understanding of what it's like to use emergency contraception and feel more informed, supported, and empowered in your own decisions.

Chapter 13

Regulatory and Approval History

"How did ulipristal acetate and Plan B make their way to the pharmacy shelves? Understanding their development and approval journey helps shine a light on the challenges and triumphs of making emergency contraception available worldwide."

The journey of **emergency contraceptives** from the lab to the pharmacy shelf has been a long and complex one, marked by both medical advances and societal debates. The stories of **Plan B** and **ulipristal acetate** are not just about science; they are also about **advocacy, policy changes**, and the struggle to make reproductive health accessible to all. Understanding the **regulatory and approval history** of these medications reveals the hurdles that had to be overcome to bring them into the hands of those who need them, as well as the progress that's been made in ensuring broader availability.

Plan B, one of the first emergency contraceptives to be widely available, was developed as a **levonorgestrel-based** option designed to prevent pregnancy after unprotected sex. Initially, emergency contraception was available only through healthcare providers, often making it difficult for those in need to access it promptly. Plan B was first approved by the **U.S. Food and Drug Administration (FDA) in 1999**, but it was available only with a prescription. This limitation posed a significant barrier for those needing timely access, as the effectiveness of Plan B decreases the longer it takes to administer after unprotected intercourse.

The path to making Plan B available **over the counter** was a major milestone, but it wasn't without its obstacles. The move faced significant **political and social resistance**, with opponents arguing about the moral implications of making emergency contraception easily accessible to younger individuals. After years of advocacy by health organizations, scientists, and women's rights groups, the FDA finally approved Plan B for **over-the-counter** use for individuals aged **18 and older** in **2006**. In **2009**, the age restriction was lowered to **17**, and by **2013**, after legal battles and mounting public pressure, Plan B was made available **without a prescription** for individuals of all ages. This was a landmark decision that improved access and allowed people to obtain emergency contraception without needing to consult a healthcare provider.

Ulipristal acetate, marketed as **Ella**, entered the scene later, providing another option for emergency contraception with a longer window of effectiveness. **Ulipristal acetate** was developed as a **selective progesterone receptor modulator** (SPRM), allowing it to delay ovulation more effectively than Plan B, even in the later stages of the menstrual cycle. It was first approved by the **European Medicines Agency (EMA)** in **2009** and by the **FDA** in **2010**.

Unlike Plan B, ulipristal acetate was approved as a **prescription-only** medication in the United States, a status that remains in place today. This requirement for a prescription, while ensuring medical oversight, also introduces barriers to quick access—something that has sparked ongoing debates among healthcare advocates.

The approval processes for both **Plan B** and **ulipristal acetate** were shaped not only by scientific research but also by **public opinion**, **ethical debates**, and **political pressures**. The initial pushback against emergency contraception was largely influenced by misconceptions about its mechanism of action, with many opponents erroneously claiming that these medications induced abortion. Advocacy groups had to work tirelessly to educate both the public and policymakers about the true nature of these drugs—that they work by preventing pregnancy, not terminating it.

The **global regulatory landscape** for emergency contraception has been similarly diverse and complex. In some countries, emergency contraceptives have been readily embraced, with both **ulipristal acetate** and **Plan B** available either over the counter or by prescription. In other regions, access remains highly restricted, often due to cultural or religious beliefs that frame the use of emergency contraception as morally unacceptable. In countries where reproductive health rights are politically contested, the availability of these medications can be limited by law, meaning that individuals in need of emergency contraception may face significant barriers to access.

One of the key **triumphs** in the journey of these medications has been the role of **nonprofit organisations** and **public health initiatives**. Groups like **Planned Parenthood**, **Women on Waves**, and various **international health NGOs** have played crucial roles in expanding access to emergency contraception worldwide. They have not only advocated for regulatory changes but also provided education and distributed emergency contraceptives in regions where access is otherwise restricted. Their efforts have helped millions of people obtain the care they need, empowering them with more control over their reproductive health.

Another major development in the regulatory history of emergency contraception has been the rise of **online pharmacies** and **telehealth services**, which have changed how people access medications like **ulipristal acetate**. In countries where prescriptions are required, telehealth has made it easier for people to obtain a prescription without needing to visit a doctor in person. This shift has been especially beneficial during the **COVID-19 pandemic**, which saw increased reliance on remote healthcare solutions, making it easier for individuals to obtain emergency contraception from the safety of their homes.

However, despite progress, challenges remain. The regulatory history of emergency contraceptives continues to evolve, influenced by ongoing debates about reproductive rights, healthcare accessibility, and the role of government in regulating personal health choices. In some places, the approval of **over-the-counter access** remains stalled, and misinformation about the safety and effectiveness of emergency contraception still persists, preventing individuals from making informed decisions.

By understanding the **regulatory and approval history** of **ulipristal acetate** and **Plan B**, we gain insight into the broader struggles and successes that have shaped the availability of these crucial medications. The journey to make emergency contraception accessible has been marked by setbacks, but also by significant victories that have improved reproductive health for millions around the world. It's a testament to the importance of **advocacy**, **education**, and the ongoing fight for reproductive rights.

As we explore the history of these medications, we're reminded of the many voices—scientists, healthcare providers, advocates, and individuals—who have worked tirelessly to ensure that emergency contraception is an option available to those who need it. Their efforts highlight the importance of continued progress, ensuring that emergency contraception is not only safe and effective but also readily available to everyone, regardless of where they live or their circumstances.

Chapter 14

Future of Emergency Contraception

"The world of medicine is always evolving. What's on the horizon for emergency contraception? From new innovations to future research directions, discover what's next for preventing pregnancy when it matters most."

The story of **emergency contraception** is not over. As science and technology continue to advance, so too do the possibilities for improving the ways we prevent unintended pregnancies. With both **ulipristal acetate** and **Plan B** providing effective options today, researchers and healthcare professionals are looking to the future, exploring new innovations, expanding accessibility, and addressing the challenges that remain. In this chapter, we will explore the potential future developments in emergency contraception, considering what might lie ahead for both the technology and the individuals who rely on it.

One of the most promising areas of research is the **development of new molecules** that could enhance the effectiveness of emergency contraception, potentially extending the window of use beyond the current five-day limit of **ulipristal acetate**. Scientists are also working to develop **multi-functional contraceptives**—drugs that can act as emergency contraception while providing additional health benefits, such as protection against sexually transmitted infections (STIs). Such multi-functional pills could provide a broader approach to reproductive health, addressing more needs with a single solution.

Another important area of focus for the future is improving **efficacy for all body types**. While **Plan B** and **ulipristal acetate** have proven effective, research suggests that **body weight** can significantly impact their success rates, particularly for those with a higher **Body Mass Index (BMI)**. Future emergency contraceptives might be developed with **formulations** that maintain high efficacy across a wider range of body weights, ensuring that all individuals can rely on them with the same confidence. Understanding the biological mechanisms behind weight-related efficacy differences could lead to innovations that make emergency contraception universally effective, regardless of body composition.

Long-term contraceptive solutions that can be administered on an as-needed basis are also being considered. Imagine a **contraceptive implant** or a **patch** that could be activated when needed—offering the benefits of immediate action like emergency contraception but with the ease of having it on hand at all times. Such technologies would bridge the gap between long-term contraception and emergency methods, providing flexibility and control without the urgency of obtaining a medication after unprotected intercourse.

There is also growing interest in developing **non-hormonal emergency contraceptives**. Both Plan B and ulipristal acetate work by affecting hormone levels to prevent pregnancy, which can lead to side effects such as **nausea**, **headaches**, and **menstrual changes**. Non-hormonal options could offer a way to avoid these side effects, making emergency contraception more comfortable for those who are sensitive to hormonal changes. Researchers are exploring **enzyme inhibitors** and **novel chemical compounds** that could prevent fertilisation without altering the body's natural hormonal balance. Such advancements could transform the landscape of emergency contraception by offering highly effective, hormone-free alternatives.

Accessibility is another critical frontier for the future of emergency contraception. As telehealth and **digital healthcare** solutions continue to grow, the hope is that emergency contraception will become easier to obtain, regardless of location. In areas where access to pharmacies or healthcare providers is limited, innovations like **online consultations, mail-order pharmacies**, and even **mobile health units** could bring emergency contraception to those who currently face barriers. The goal is to eliminate the logistical hurdles that prevent people from getting timely access to emergency contraception when they need it most.

Education and awareness campaigns are also expected to evolve, leveraging digital platforms to ensure that more people have accurate information about emergency contraception. Misconceptions about the safety, effectiveness, and ethical considerations of emergency contraceptives continue to be a barrier for many. Future public health initiatives might use **social media, online influencers**, and even **virtual reality educational tools** to provide clearer, more accessible information about emergency contraception, demystifying its use and reducing stigma.

Global availability is a crucial aspect of the future of emergency contraception. While access has improved significantly in many parts of the world, there are still regions where emergency contraception is restricted or even illegal. The future of emergency contraception must include an emphasis on making these medications available to everyone, regardless of their geographical location. International health organizations are working to remove **regulatory barriers** and advocate for the widespread availability of emergency contraceptives, ensuring that reproductive health options are a fundamental right for all individuals.

Male contraceptives are another area with promising implications for emergency contraception. Currently, the responsibility for emergency contraception largely falls on individuals who can become pregnant. However, the development of effective **male contraceptives** could significantly change this dynamic, providing more options for couples to share responsibility for preventing unintended pregnancies. Although research into male contraception is still in the early stages, future developments could provide new, shared methods that further empower individuals in their reproductive choices.

Artificial intelligence (AI) and **personalized medicine** also have roles to play in the future of emergency contraception. Imagine an AI-powered app that could predict your ovulation cycle with greater precision, helping you determine the most effective time to use emergency contraception. Advances in **genetic research** and personalized healthcare might also lead to emergency contraceptives that are tailored to your unique biology, maximizing effectiveness while minimizing side effects. These innovations represent the cutting edge of reproductive health technology, offering hope for more customized and effective emergency contraceptive options.

In this chapter, we'll also consider the **societal and legal landscape** that will shape the future of emergency contraception. As the conversation around **reproductive rights** continues to evolve, so too will the policies that govern access to emergency contraceptives. The hope is that, in the future, emergency contraception will be viewed as an essential aspect of healthcare, with no unnecessary restrictions on who can access it or when. The ongoing advocacy efforts of reproductive rights groups, alongside the shifting political landscape, suggest that we may see even greater strides toward universal access in the coming years.

The future of emergency contraception is filled with **potential**—new drugs, improved formulations, enhanced accessibility, and innovative delivery systems all promise a more effective, inclusive, and user-friendly approach to preventing unintended pregnancies. These advancements not only aim to improve efficacy and comfort but also strive to put emergency contraception into the hands of everyone who needs it, regardless of their circumstances.

As we look ahead, it's clear that the goal is to provide even greater **control** over reproductive health, reduce the stigma associated with emergency contraception, and ensure that these medications are available to all individuals who need them. The innovations on the horizon reflect the ongoing commitment to empowering people through better, safer, and more accessible reproductive health options. In the future, emergency contraception won't just be about preventing pregnancy—it will be about offering greater freedom, choice, and confidence in managing one's reproductive health, no matter the situation.

Chapter 15

A Practical Guide to Using Emergency Contraception

"When the moment comes, you want to know exactly what to do. This practical guide provides a step-by-step look at obtaining and using ulipristal acetate and Plan B—so you can be confident in your emergency contraception choice."

Emergency contraception is all about quick, decisive action during unexpected situations. Whether a condom breaks, you forget to take your regular birth control, or any other mishap occurs, knowing how to proceed with **ulipristal acetate** or **Plan B** is crucial. When the need arises, having a clear guide can help you avoid panic, make the right choice, and use these emergency contraceptives effectively. This chapter is designed to provide you with that **step-by-step roadmap**.

The first thing you need to know is **how to assess your options** based on timing. **Plan B** and **ulipristal acetate** both work to prevent pregnancy, but they are most effective when used within specific timeframes. **Plan B** is best used within **72 hours (3 days)** of unprotected intercourse, while **ulipristal acetate** can be taken up to **120 hours (5 days)** after, with consistent effectiveness. The sooner you take either medication, the better it will work. The key is to determine where you are in your timeline and choose accordingly.

Step 1: Deciding Which Emergency Contraceptive to Use

- **If it's been less than 72 hours** since the incident, **Plan B** can be an effective choice, especially if you can easily access a pharmacy without delay.
- **If it's been more than 72 hours but less than 120 hours**, or if you're unsure about your cycle and think ovulation might be close,

ulipristal acetate is generally the better choice for extended effectiveness.
- **Body weight** can also influence your decision. For individuals with a **higher BMI**, ulipristal acetate tends to maintain its effectiveness better than Plan B, which might be less effective in people weighing over **165 pounds (75 kg)**.

Step 2: Obtaining the Medication

- **Plan B** can often be purchased **over-the-counter** at most pharmacies. In many locations, you don't need a prescription or even to interact with a pharmacist—it's available off the shelf.
- **Ulipristal acetate**, on the other hand, usually requires a **prescription**. You can obtain a prescription from your healthcare provider or through a **telehealth service**, which can expedite the process if you need it urgently.

- Consider **telehealth services** if you cannot access a healthcare provider in person or if you want the convenience of an online consultation. Many online platforms can provide prescriptions and even mail the medication directly to you.

Step 3: Purchasing and Handling

- For **Plan B**, simply visit a pharmacy, a large grocery store, or even some convenience stores. It's available without age restrictions, but availability may vary by location.
- **Ulipristal acetate** will require picking up your prescription from a pharmacy, or you can opt for **online pharmacies** that deliver the medication to your door. Make sure to double-check any delivery timelines if you choose to order online.

Step 4: Taking the Medication

- **Take the pill as soon as possible** once you have it in your possession. **Timing is everything**—the sooner you take it after unprotected intercourse, the higher its chances of working effectively.
- **Take the pill with water**, and you may want to have a light snack to help avoid **nausea**, a common side effect. If you vomit within **two hours** of taking the pill, contact your healthcare provider to determine if you need a replacement dose.

Step 5: Managing Side Effects

- Expect possible side effects such as **nausea**, **dizziness**, **headache**, **fatigue**, or **changes in your next period**. Your period might come earlier or later than expected, and it may be heavier or lighter. These side effects are usually mild and short-lived, but being prepared can help you handle them calmly.

- Keep **hydrated** and consider **resting** if you feel tired or nauseous. These symptoms typically resolve in a day or two.

Step 6: Monitoring Your Menstrual Cycle

- **Track your period** after taking the emergency contraceptive. Your next cycle might be a little off schedule—if your period is more than a week late, it's a good idea to take a **pregnancy test**. While these medications are effective, no method is foolproof, and it's always best to confirm.

Step 7: Planning for the Future

- **Emergency contraception** should be seen as a backup plan, not a primary method of birth control. If you find yourself needing it more than once, it might be time to discuss **long-term contraceptive options** with your healthcare provider. They can help you find a method that works well for you, reducing the

likelihood of needing emergency contraception again.
- Options like **birth control pills**, **IUDs**, **implants**, or **contraceptive patches** offer more consistent protection and reduce the stress of repeated emergency situations.

Additional Considerations

- If you're feeling **anxious** about purchasing emergency contraception in person, many online pharmacies provide **discreet packaging** and delivery, allowing you to receive the medication without concerns about privacy.
- If you're in a **rural area** or somewhere where pharmacies may not carry these medications readily, consider looking into **online pharmacies** in advance. Knowing your options before an emergency arises can make all the difference when you need to act quickly.

Handling Special Situations

- **If the pharmacy is out of stock**, consider going to a different pharmacy or asking if they can recommend another nearby location that has it available. Alternatively, if you're opting for ulipristal acetate, check with telehealth services to see if they can assist you.
- If you're **travelling**, emergency contraception may be more challenging to obtain due to local regulations or availability issues. Plan ahead by checking the regulations in your destination and consider bringing emergency contraception with you if it's legally permitted.

By understanding each of these steps—**deciding, obtaining, taking, and managing**—you can approach the need for emergency contraception with more confidence and less stress. When faced with an unexpected situation, knowing exactly what to do and where to go is empowering. This practical guide is here to ensure you have everything you need to make informed, prompt decisions for your reproductive health, providing you with the tools to use **ulipristal acetate** or **Plan B** safely and effectively.

Conclusion

"Choosing emergency contraception is an important decision that should come with understanding and confidence. As we conclude, reflect on what you've learned about ulipristal acetate and Plan B—and feel empowered to make informed, responsible choices for your reproductive health."

Throughout this journey, we've delved deeply into the world of **emergency contraception**—its history, its mechanisms, and the many factors that influence its effectiveness. We began with understanding the crucial role of emergency contraception in managing reproductive health, particularly in those moments when life doesn't go according to plan. Whether it was an unexpected contraceptive failure or a moment of uncertainty, having a clear understanding of your options is empowering.

Ulipristal acetate and **Plan B** are two key players in this landscape, and each has its own unique set of strengths. **Plan B**, with its over-the-counter availability and easy accessibility, provides a fast, reliable backup option when time is of the essence. On the other hand, **ulipristal acetate** offers a longer window of effectiveness, remaining a solid option for up to **five days** after unprotected intercourse and maintaining higher efficacy close to ovulation. Knowing these differences gives you the power to choose what works best for you based on your specific situation.

We explored the **science behind how these medications work**—from their mechanisms of action in delaying ovulation to how they interact with different body types and health conditions. Understanding the way these drugs function helps demystify the process, making it easier to see them as effective, reliable tools rather than something to be feared or misunderstood. We've also discussed the **impact of body weight**, timing, and other medications, emphasizing how these factors can influence the success of emergency contraception.

Another key topic we addressed was the **availability and accessibility** of ulipristal acetate and Plan B. For many people, the ability to obtain emergency contraception quickly is critical, and the journey of making these medications accessible has been fraught with challenges, both regulatory and cultural. The evolution of access—from prescription-only to over-the-counter availability—represents significant progress, but it's also a reminder that reproductive healthcare access is still an ongoing battle in many parts of the world.

We confronted the **myths and misconceptions** surrounding emergency contraception, dispelling misinformation about these drugs being forms of abortion or causing long-term damage. Knowing the truth about emergency contraception is vital to making informed decisions and reducing the stigma that still surrounds their use. It's about reclaiming control over your reproductive health and understanding that using emergency contraception is a responsible choice when things don't go as planned.

Personal stories provided real insight into the human experience of using emergency contraception—highlighting the emotional complexities, challenges, and victories that come with making such decisions. Whether it was someone navigating the anxiety of a missed period or figuring out how to obtain a prescription while travelling, these narratives brought to life the very real situations where emergency contraception is a necessary, empowering choice.

We also explored the **regulatory and approval history** of these medications, appreciating the tireless efforts of advocates and healthcare providers who fought to make emergency contraception available to all. Their work reminds us that these options were hard-won, and that continued advocacy is essential for ensuring that all individuals, regardless of location or circumstance, can access the reproductive healthcare they need.

Looking to the **future**, we considered how **emergency contraception** might evolve—from new formulations and non-hormonal options to greater inclusivity through global availability and male contraceptives. The future holds promise for a more comprehensive approach to emergency contraception, one that is accessible, effective, and tailored to the needs of diverse populations. Advances in technology and personalised medicine could pave the way for even more effective, comfortable options, ensuring that everyone has the tools they need to protect their reproductive health.

In the **practical guide** provided in Chapter 15, we aimed to equip you with the steps necessary to act decisively and confidently in times of need. Knowing exactly what to do—from deciding which medication to choose to understanding how to obtain and take it—can make an overwhelming situation far more manageable. Emergency contraception is about taking control when things don't go as planned, and having a practical plan in place is key to ensuring you're ready if and when the time comes.

As we close this book, remember that **emergency contraception** is about giving yourself the power to make choices for your body and your future. It is about **responsibility**, **empowerment**, and taking charge of your reproductive health when faced with the unexpected. **Ulipristal acetate** and **Plan B** are both effective and reliable options, each suited to different circumstances, and the knowledge you now have can guide you in choosing what works best for you.

Your reproductive health is your own, and making informed decisions about it is a right that everyone deserves. By understanding how emergency contraception works, dispelling myths, navigating the practicalities, and appreciating the ongoing efforts to expand access, you are better equipped to make confident, informed choices when it comes to preventing an unplanned pregnancy.

Whether this knowledge is for yourself or to help guide a loved one, you now have the information needed to use **emergency contraception** wisely and effectively. Emergencies are never predictable, but with the right knowledge and tools, you can face them head-on with confidence and control. The ability to make empowered choices is what true **reproductive freedom** is all about, and emergency contraception is one important part of that freedom.

Appendix

"Knowledge is power. This appendix provides answers to common questions, additional resources, and support options, helping you stay informed about emergency contraception."

The journey through understanding **emergency contraception** has covered a wide range of topics—from the mechanisms of **ulipristal acetate** and **Plan B** to navigating myths and considering the future of reproductive healthcare. But even after exploring all these aspects, it's natural to still have questions. This **appendix** is designed to serve as a quick reference guide, providing answers to frequently asked questions, additional **resources** for further reading, and support options that can assist you in making informed decisions about emergency contraception.

We begin with a list of **commonly asked questions**. These are questions that people often have when considering or using emergency contraception—such as **how soon you should take Plan B or ulipristal acetate, whether it's safe to use emergency contraception multiple times**, and **what to do if you experience certain side effects**. The goal is to give you easy access to clear, concise answers so that you can feel confident about your next steps without wading through extensive information again.

The **FAQs** also include practical advice, such as how to manage situations where the pharmacy is out of stock, what to do if you're **travelling** and need access to emergency contraception, and **how to know if the medication worked**. Having these answers readily available can help you navigate an unexpected situation calmly and effectively.

Next, the appendix provides a curated list of **resources and support organisations**. These include links to **websites, hotlines**, and **local organisations** that provide support related to emergency contraception, reproductive health, and general sexual health. Some of the resources you'll find here are:

- **Planned Parenthood**: Offers both in-person and online resources, consultations, and information on all forms of contraception.
- **Bedsider.org**: An online birth control support network that provides information about different contraception options, reminders, and a database for finding clinics near you.
- **World Health Organization (WHO)**: Resources on reproductive health and emergency contraception guidelines applicable worldwide.
- **Telehealth services** that offer **online consultations** and **prescriptions** for emergency contraception, making it more convenient to access ulipristal acetate when needed.

These resources are designed to ensure you have **continuous access** to accurate information and support, whether you are facing an urgent situation or simply want to be prepared for the future. We've also included information on **how to find emergency contraception internationally**, as availability and regulations vary greatly by country. Understanding these differences can be critical if you're travelling or living abroad.

The appendix also offers a **glossary of key terms** related to emergency contraception. This section is here to demystify any technical terms or concepts you might have encountered throughout the book. Clear definitions of terms like **ovulation, pharmacokinetics, BMI, selective progesterone receptor modulator (SPRM)**, and others will help solidify your understanding of how emergency contraception works and how various factors affect its efficacy.

In addition, we've provided a **step-by-step checklist** to help you through the process of using emergency contraception effectively. This checklist includes points like:

1. **Determine which emergency contraceptive is best for your situation.**
2. **Act quickly and obtain the medication as soon as possible.**
3. **Follow instructions on when and how to take the medication.**
4. **Monitor your menstrual cycle and understand what to expect afterward.**
5. **Take a pregnancy test if your period is significantly delayed.**

Having this checklist on hand can make it easier to stay organised and ensure that no important steps are overlooked in a moment that might otherwise feel chaotic or overwhelming.

For those looking for **further reading**, we've included a list of **recommended books**, **articles**, and **scientific papers** that delve deeper into emergency contraception, reproductive health, and the social and ethical issues surrounding these topics. Whether you're a student, an educator, or simply someone who wants to explore the subject further, these resources offer additional depth and provide the context needed to understand emergency contraception from a broader perspective.

Finally, the appendix offers information on **how to talk to your healthcare provider** about emergency contraception. Many people feel uncomfortable discussing reproductive health, but having an open dialogue with your doctor or healthcare professional can ensure you receive the best care and advice. We include tips for framing your questions, discussing your contraceptive needs honestly, and ensuring you get all the information you need to make informed decisions.

The purpose of this appendix is to make sure that your journey with **emergency contraception** doesn't end with this book. **Knowledge** is the most powerful tool you have in managing your reproductive health, and this appendix is here to provide you with the information and resources you may need at any point, whether you're in an urgent situation or preparing for the future.

With these additional resources and support options, you can feel confident that you are not alone in navigating your reproductive health choices. Empowerment comes from having the right information, support, and guidance—and this appendix aims to equip you with all three, ensuring that you are informed, prepared, and ready to make the choices that are best for you.

www.ingramcontent.com/pod-product-compliance
Lightning Source LLC
Chambersburg PA
CBHW070150230526
45471CB00002B/597